MASON'S SNACK ATTACK
by Ron Henderson "The Fitness King"

This book series originated over 22 years ago with a dream to publish a children's book about a Mouse that decides to get fit and eat right along with his animal friends. Now this dream is a reality with the Mason the Mouse series.

Over the past 35 years I have been to numerous elementary schools and the one thing that seemed to be common among the children was that they liked to exercise and even more when it was fun. Now, with the increase in iPhones, iPads, the internet and so on, kids have become less active.

When my first child was born, I realized that he was more active than most kids his age—mostly because he grew up in my personal training gym and in a household that believed in the importance of taking care of one's health. With that in mind, and countless visits to area elementary schools, I was determined to write a book that would teach children the importance of moving and stretching. I am declaring to leave no child behind and crack the code on childhood obesity. When you read this book to your children they will hear about exercise and healthy eating in a fun way.

Mason's Snack Attack

ISBN-13:978-1517742669

ISBN-10:1517742668

A special thanks to my wife for her encouragement and support and to the countless children who I have spoken to over the years at various elementary schools who helped to inspire me even more to write books that would motivate children to eat healthy and exercise in a fun way.

To my first born son, Mason, who as a child spent hours in my personal training studio watching me and then when he was old enough, tried to pick up his first weight to mimic what I was doing.

I could see early on the importance of parents setting good examples in the areas of exercise and healthy eating. When people say, "Like father like son", they are more right then wrong. Even more so when we bring a child up into an environment that promotes physical activities.

Ron Henderson can be contacted at: Email baldking@gmail.com
Phone: 612-386-8178
Address: Ron Henderson

4301 Highway 7 Suite 110

St. Louis Park, MN 55416

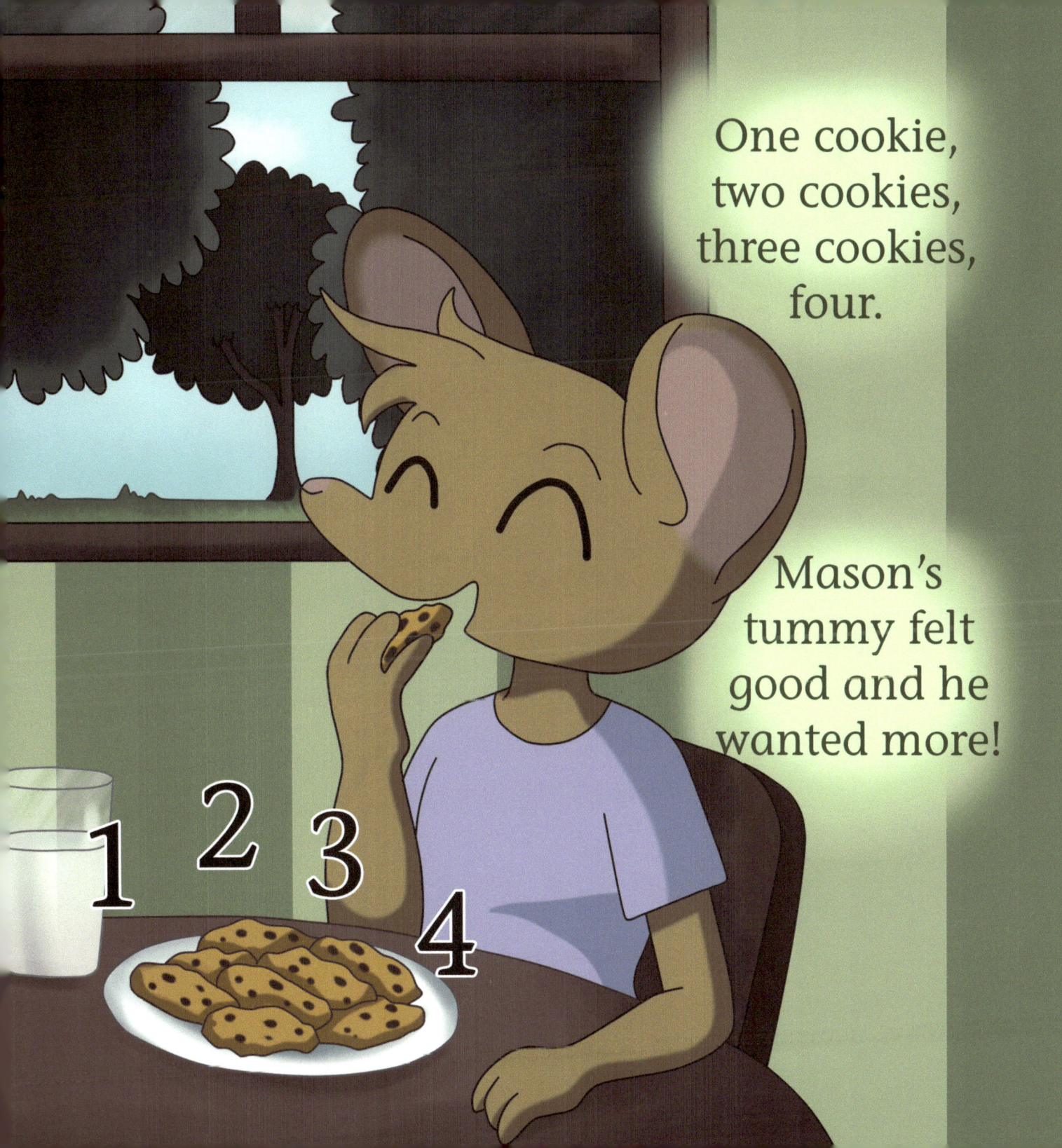

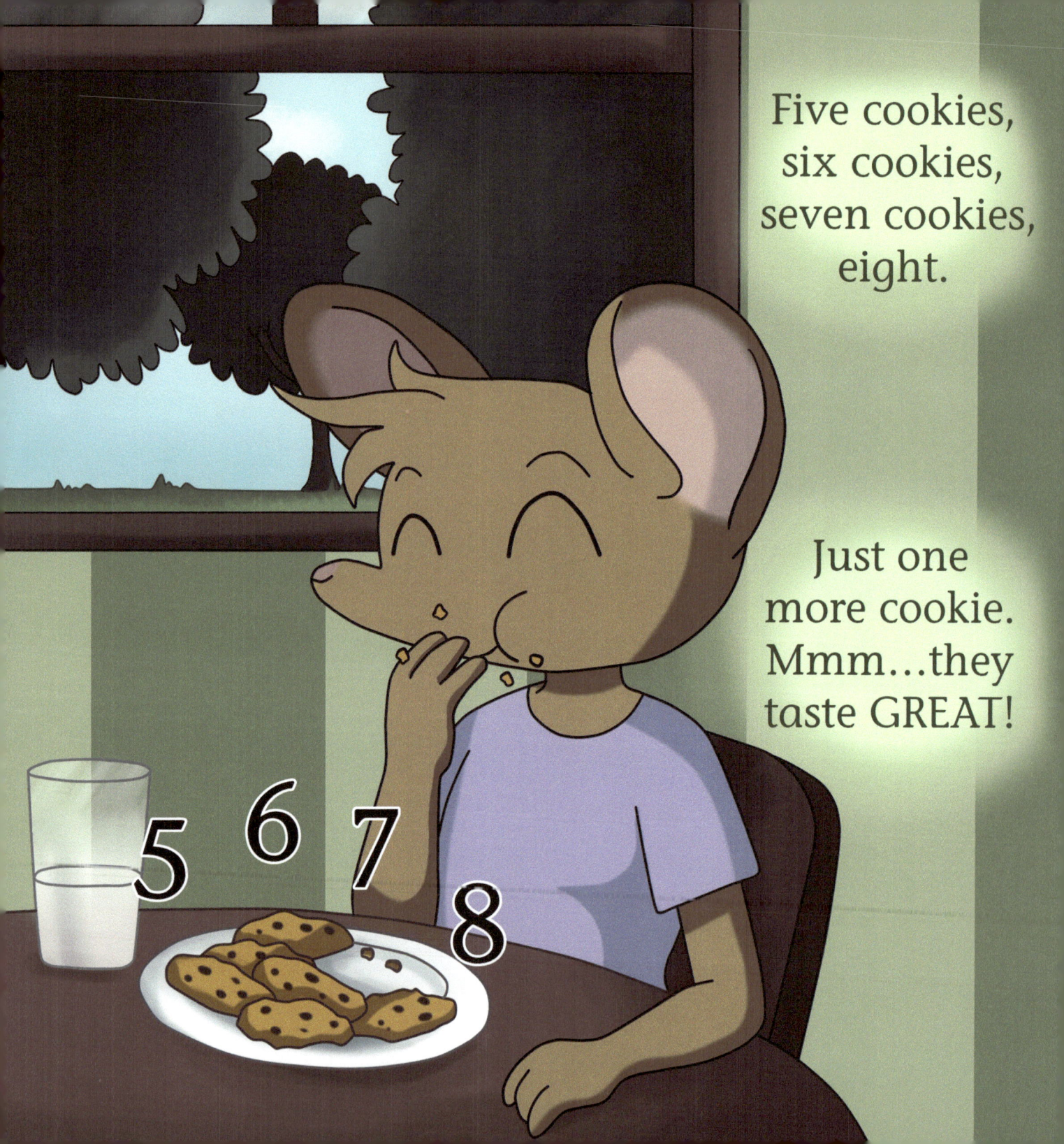

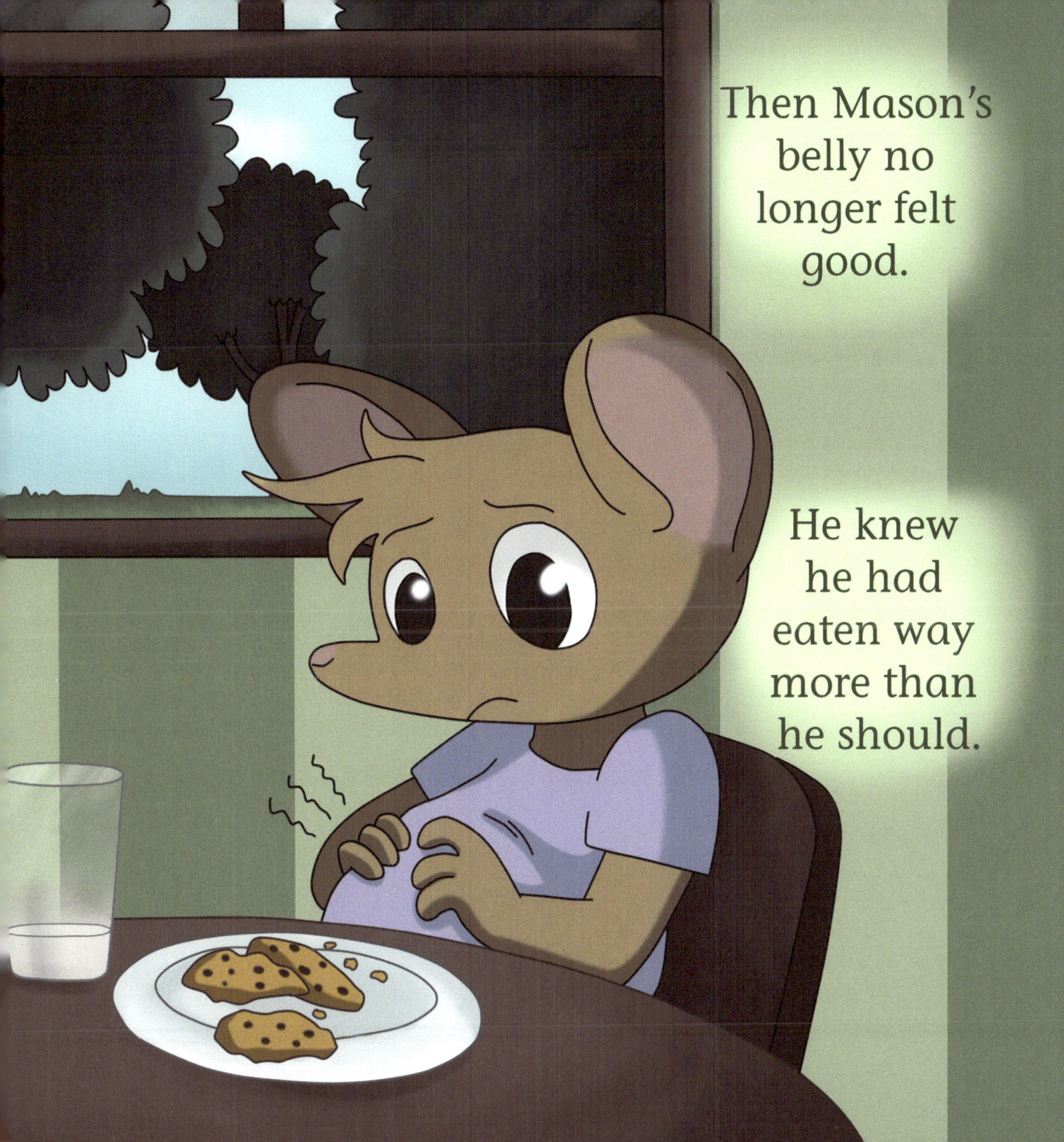

Then Mason's belly no longer felt good.

He knew he had eaten way more than he should.

Mason decided that very day to eat healthy foods and learn a new way.

"Food choices are fun! Eating better is, too! I'm excited to share what I plan to do!

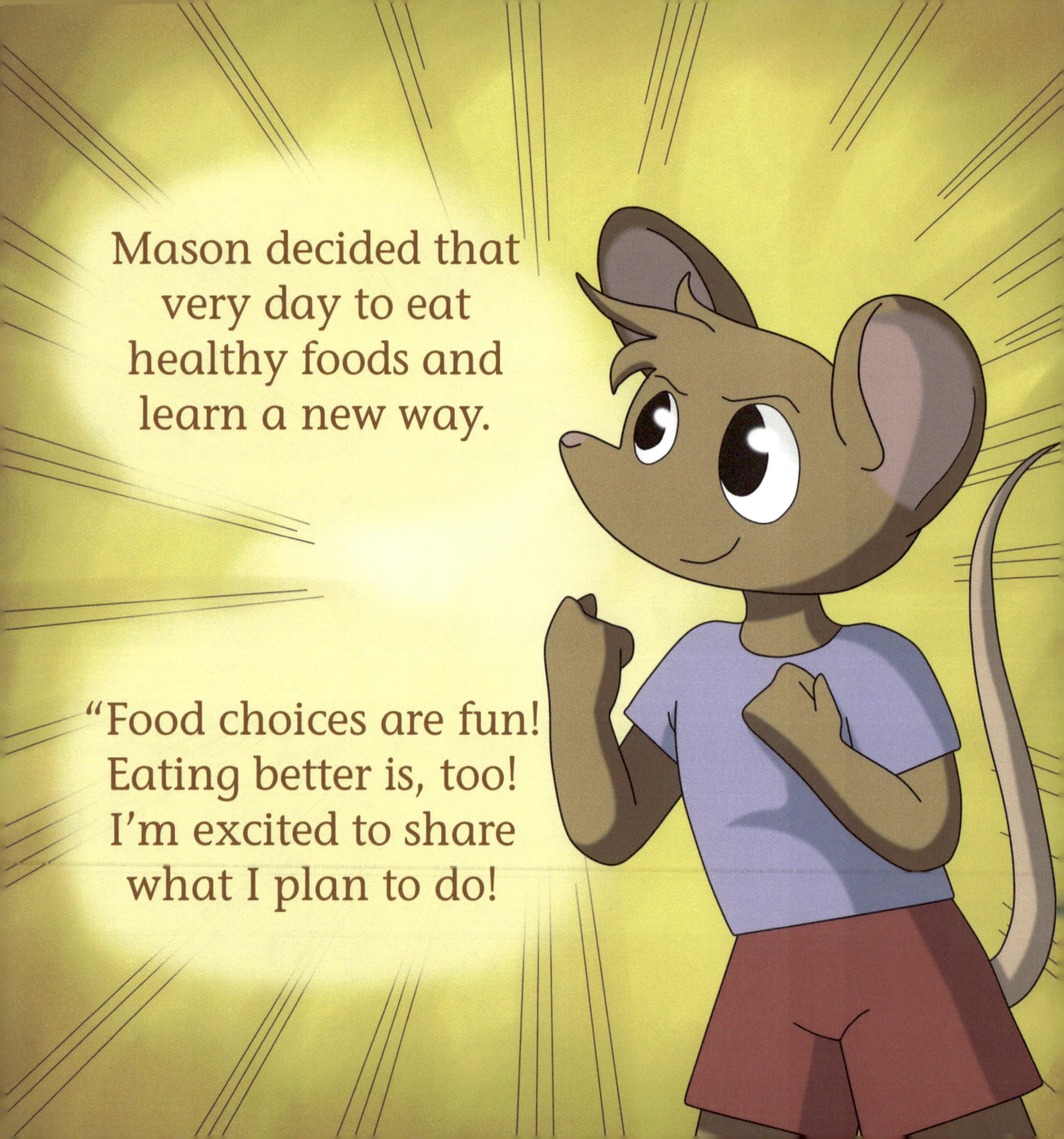

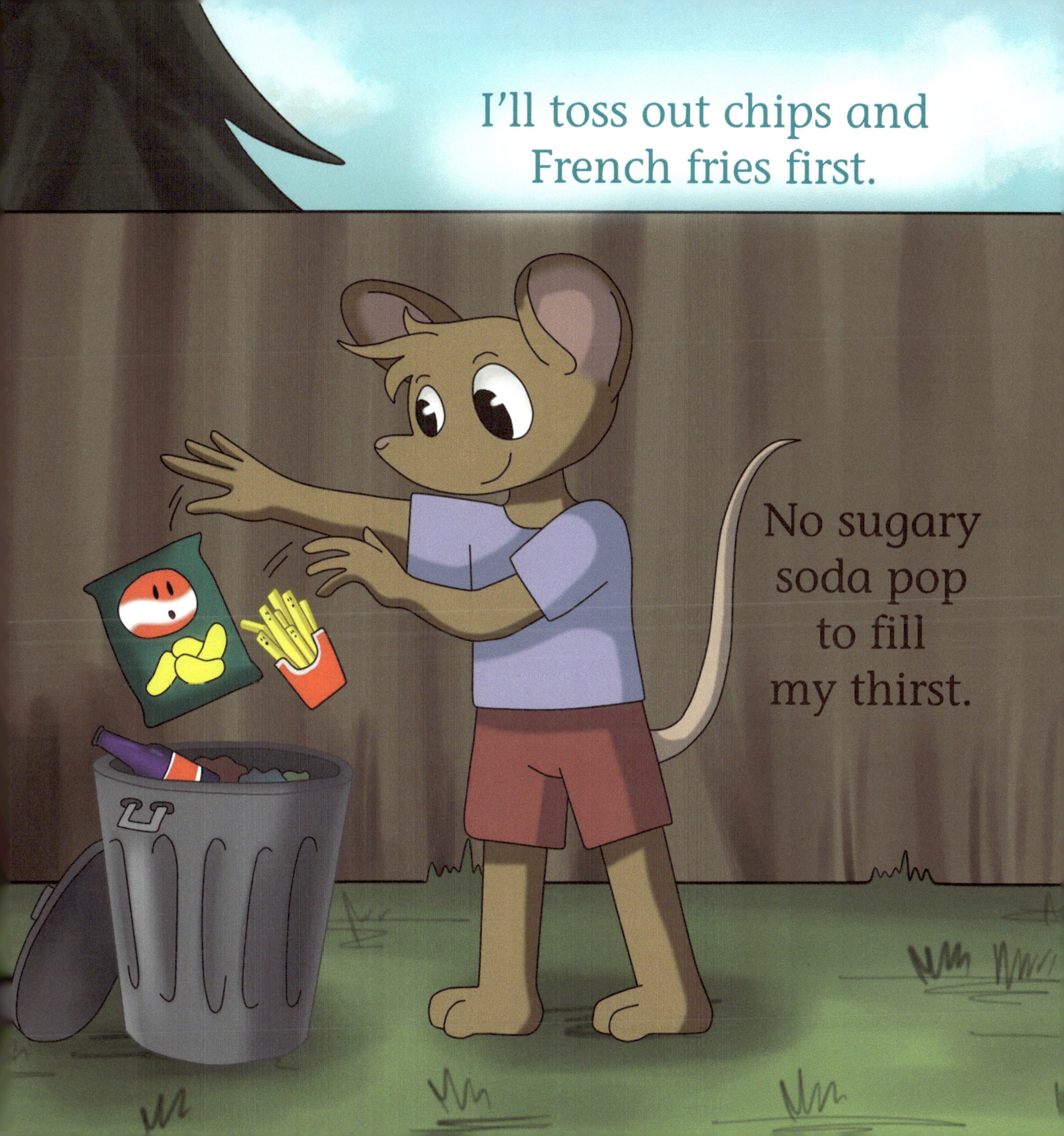

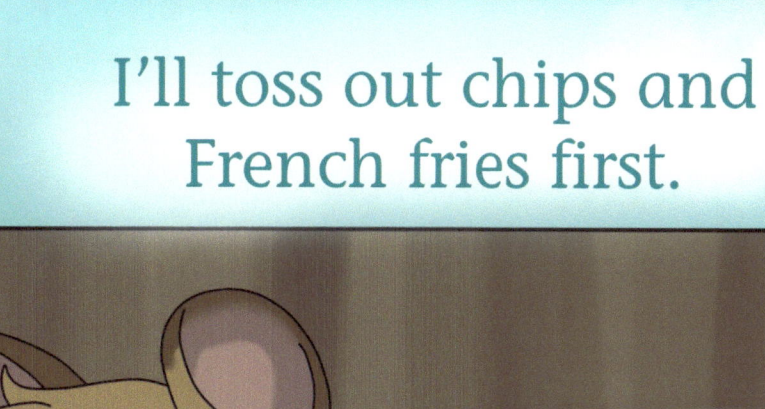

I'll toss out chips and
French fries first.

No sugary
soda pop
to fill
my thirst.

Water is the best
—clear, simple and pure.
If you are thirsty
that is the cure!

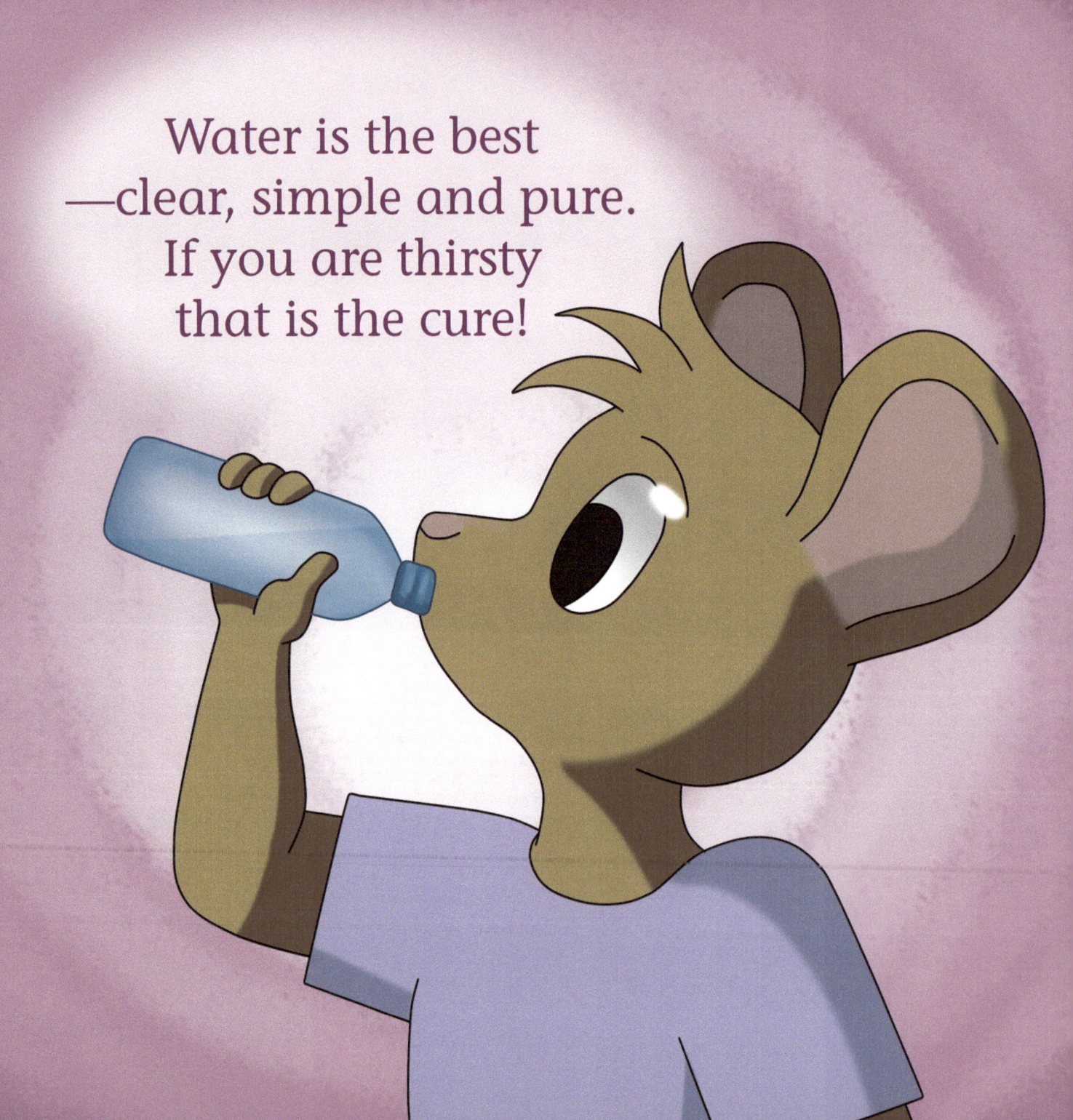

If root beer calls out to me today I will simply ignore what that sweet voice might say.

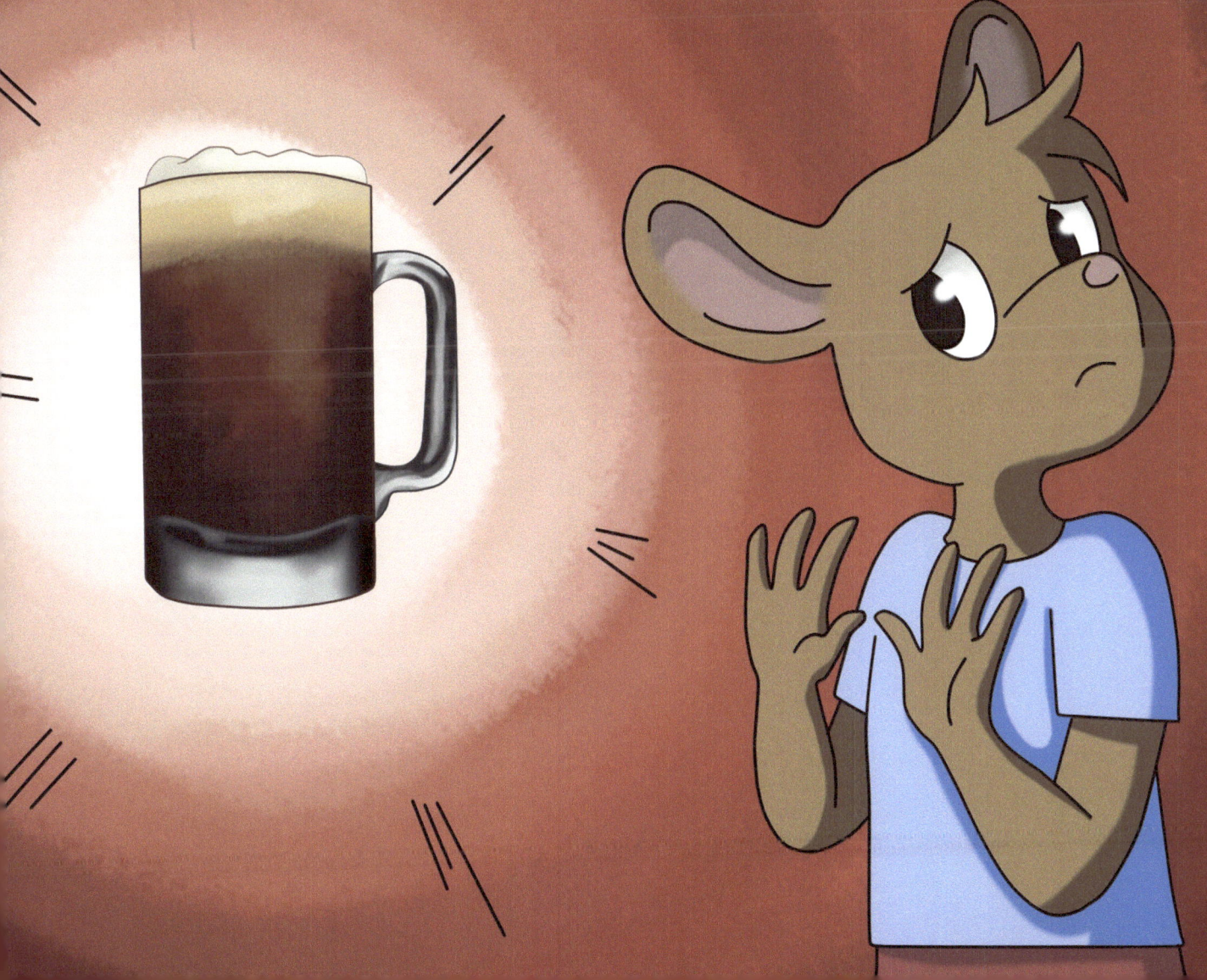

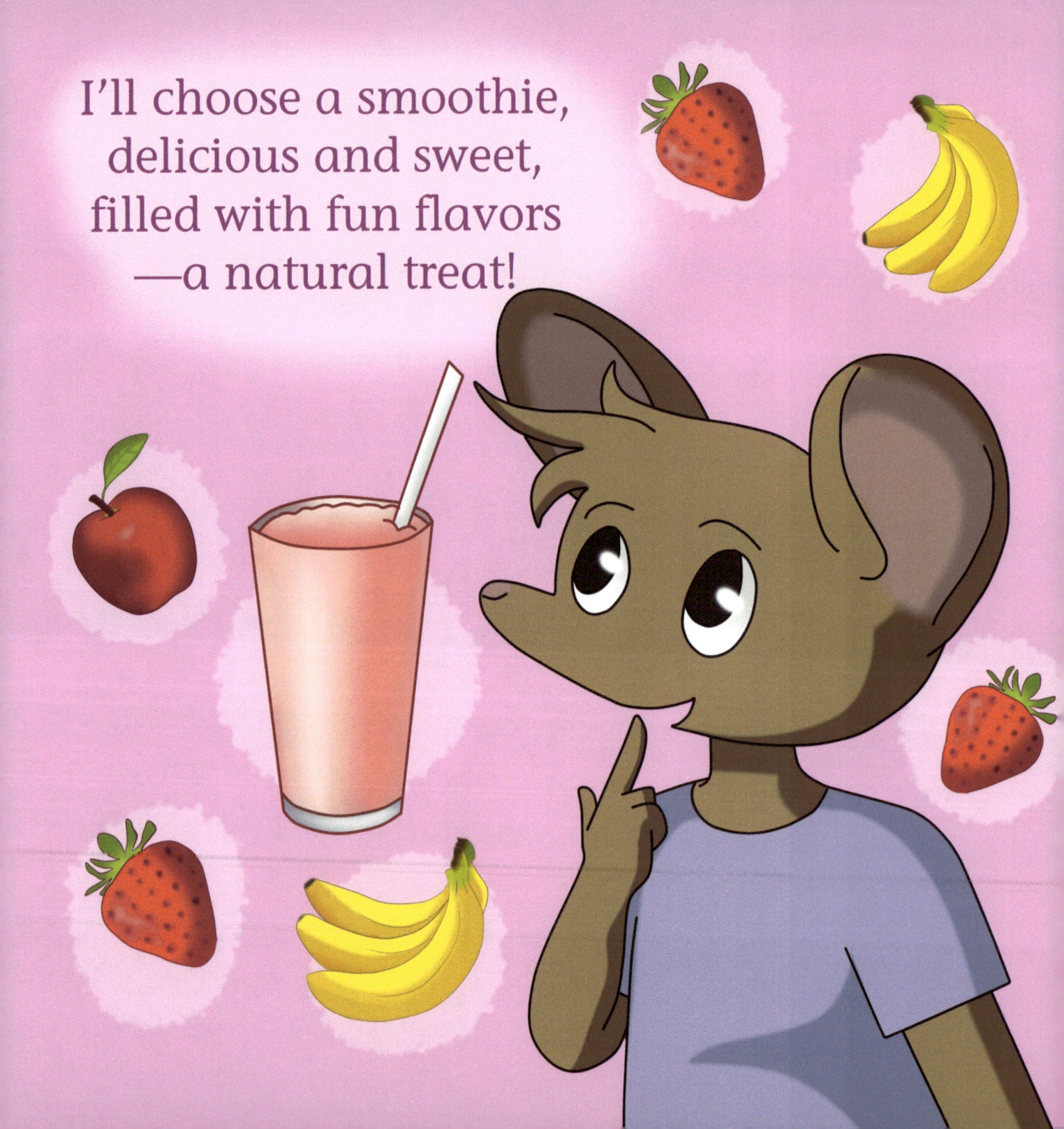

I'll choose a smoothie, delicious and sweet, filled with fun flavors —a natural treat!

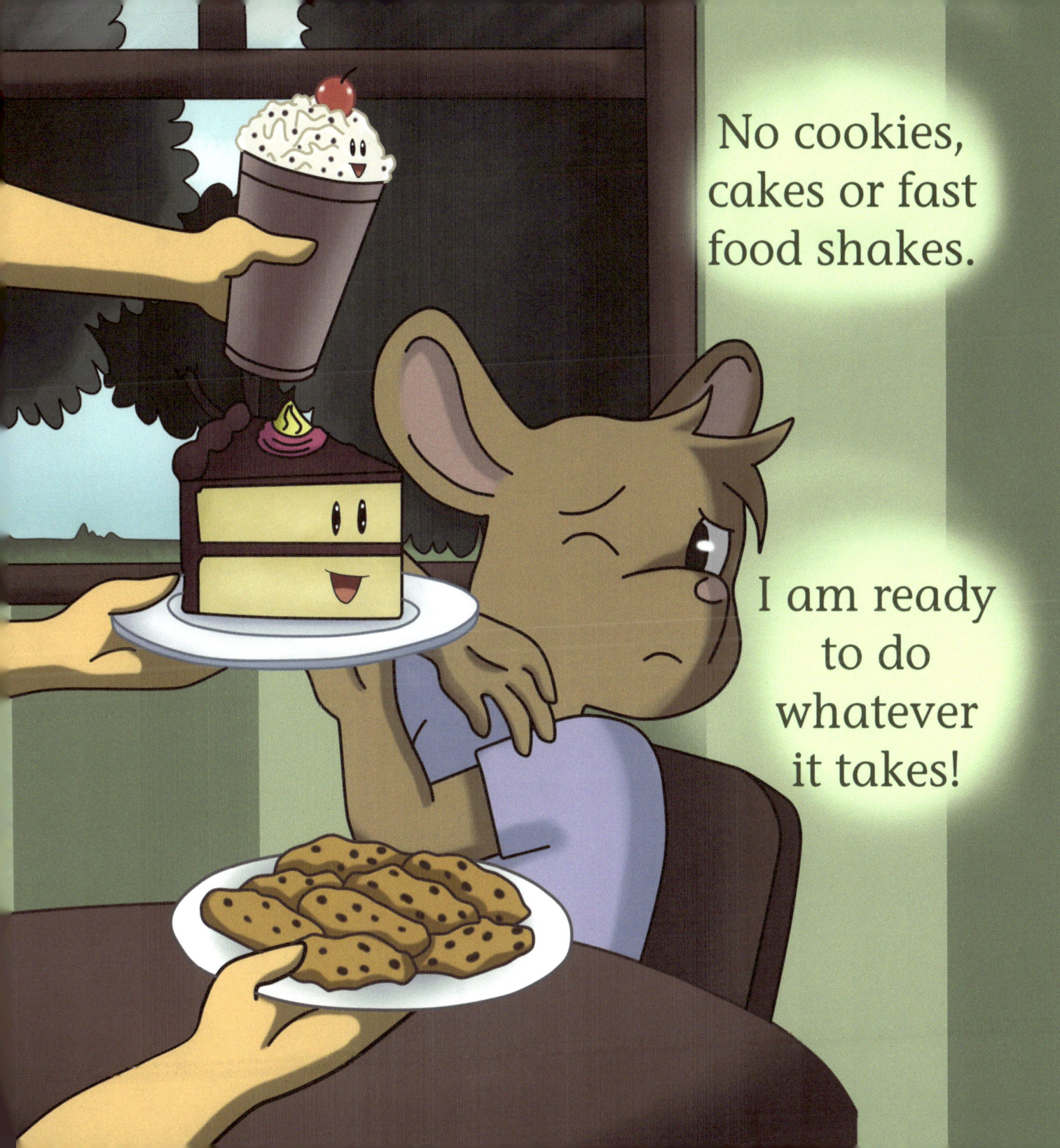

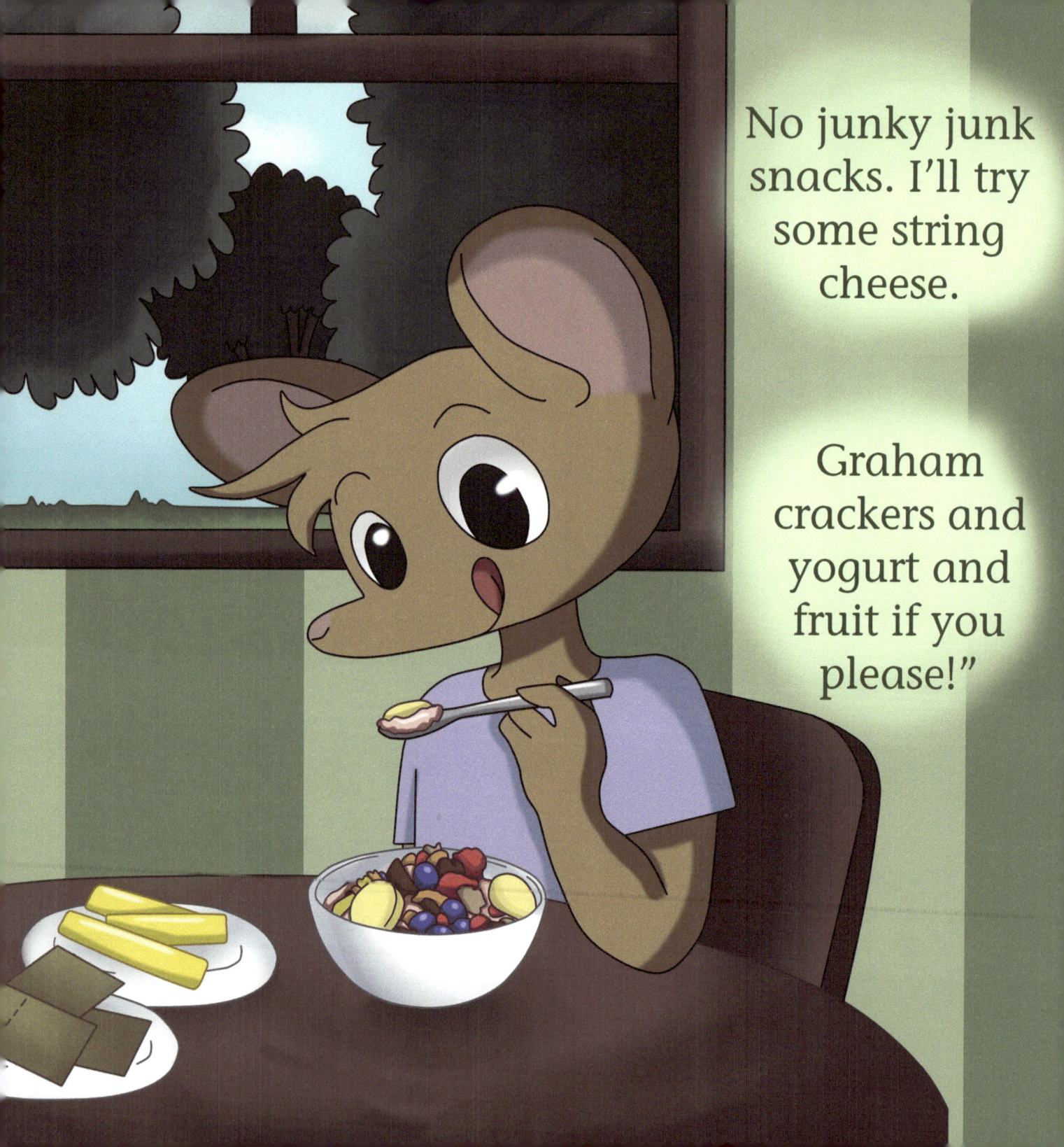

No junky junk snacks. I'll try some string cheese.

Graham crackers and yogurt and fruit if you please!"

At that very minute a thought past his mind remembering the foods that he was leaving behind.

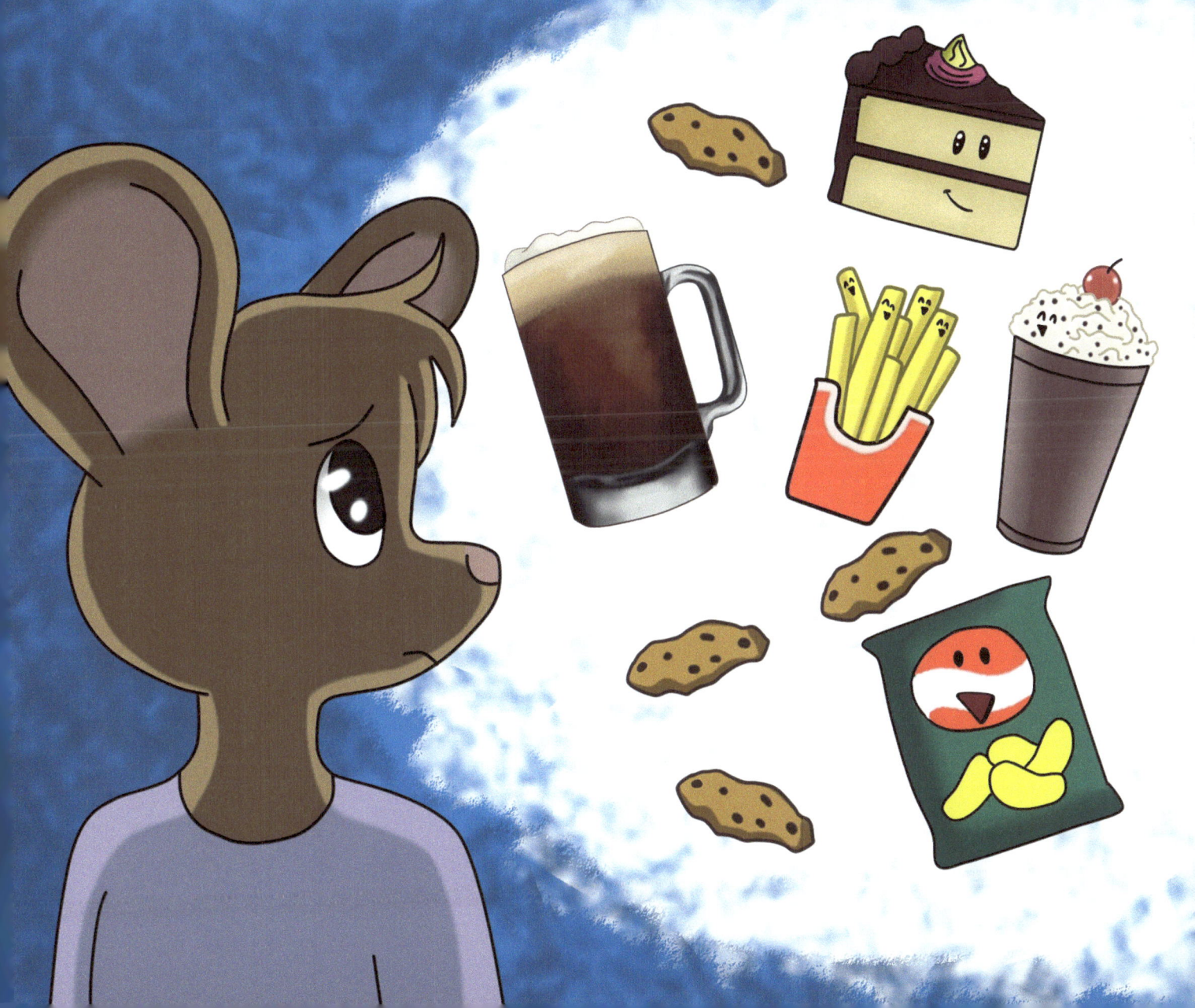

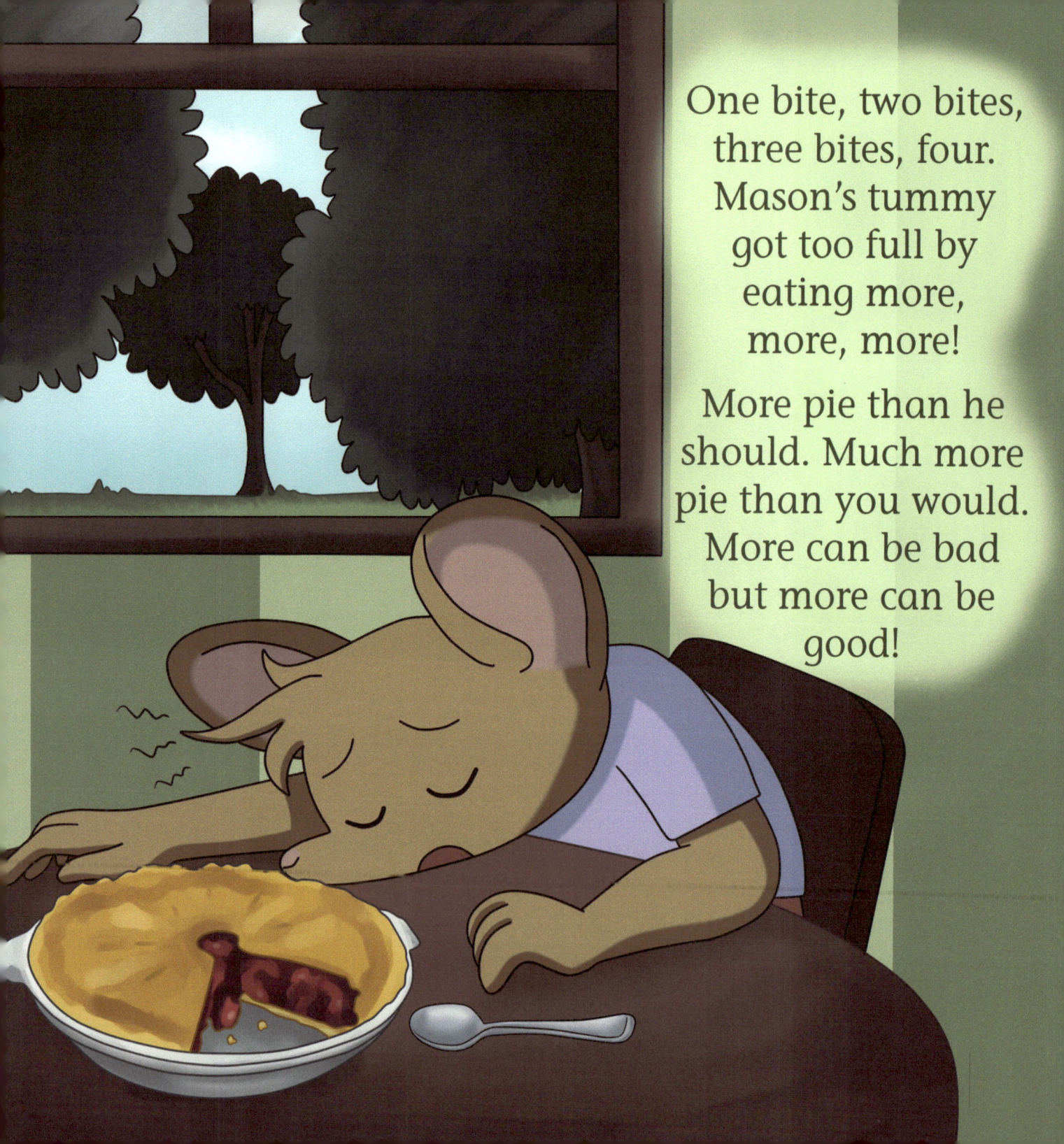

One bite, two bites, three bites, four. Mason's tummy got too full by eating more, more, more!

More pie than he should. Much more pie than you would. More can be bad but more can be good!

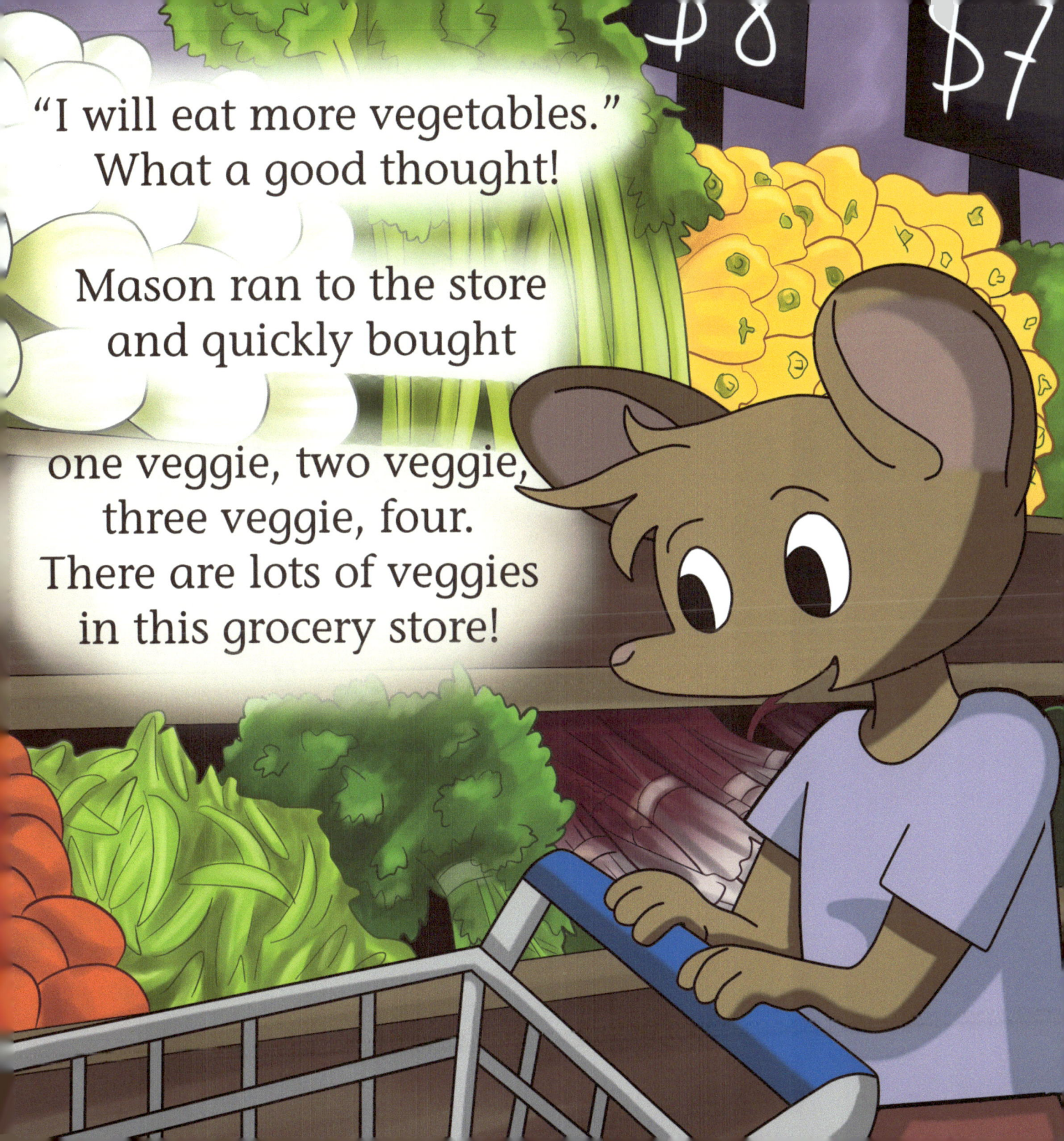

"I will eat more vegetables."
What a good thought!

Mason ran to the store
and quickly bought

one veggie, two veggie,
three veggie, four.
There are lots of veggies
in this grocery store!

From yummy asparagus to crunchy zucchini... all colors and sizes. Some large and some teeny.

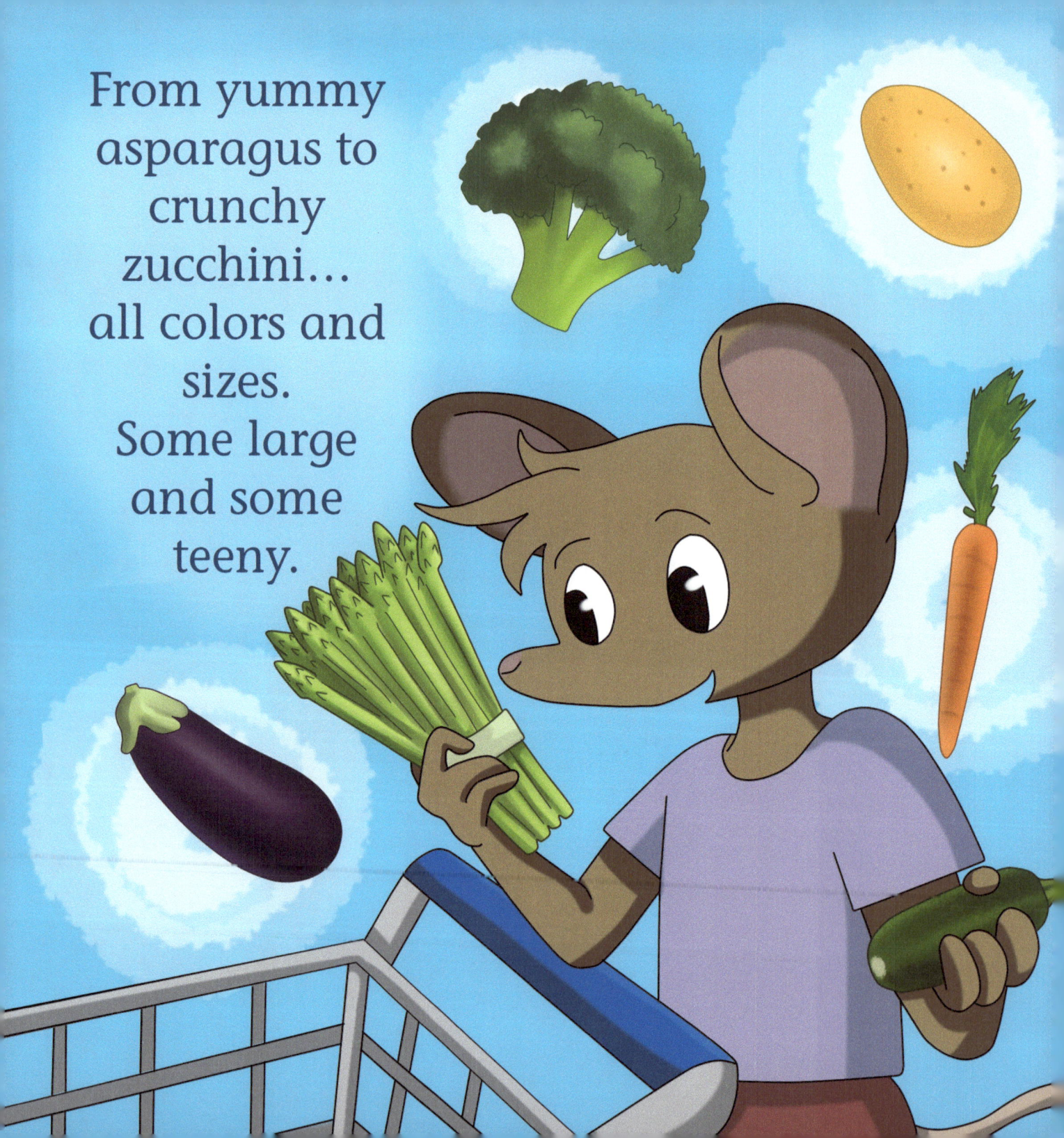

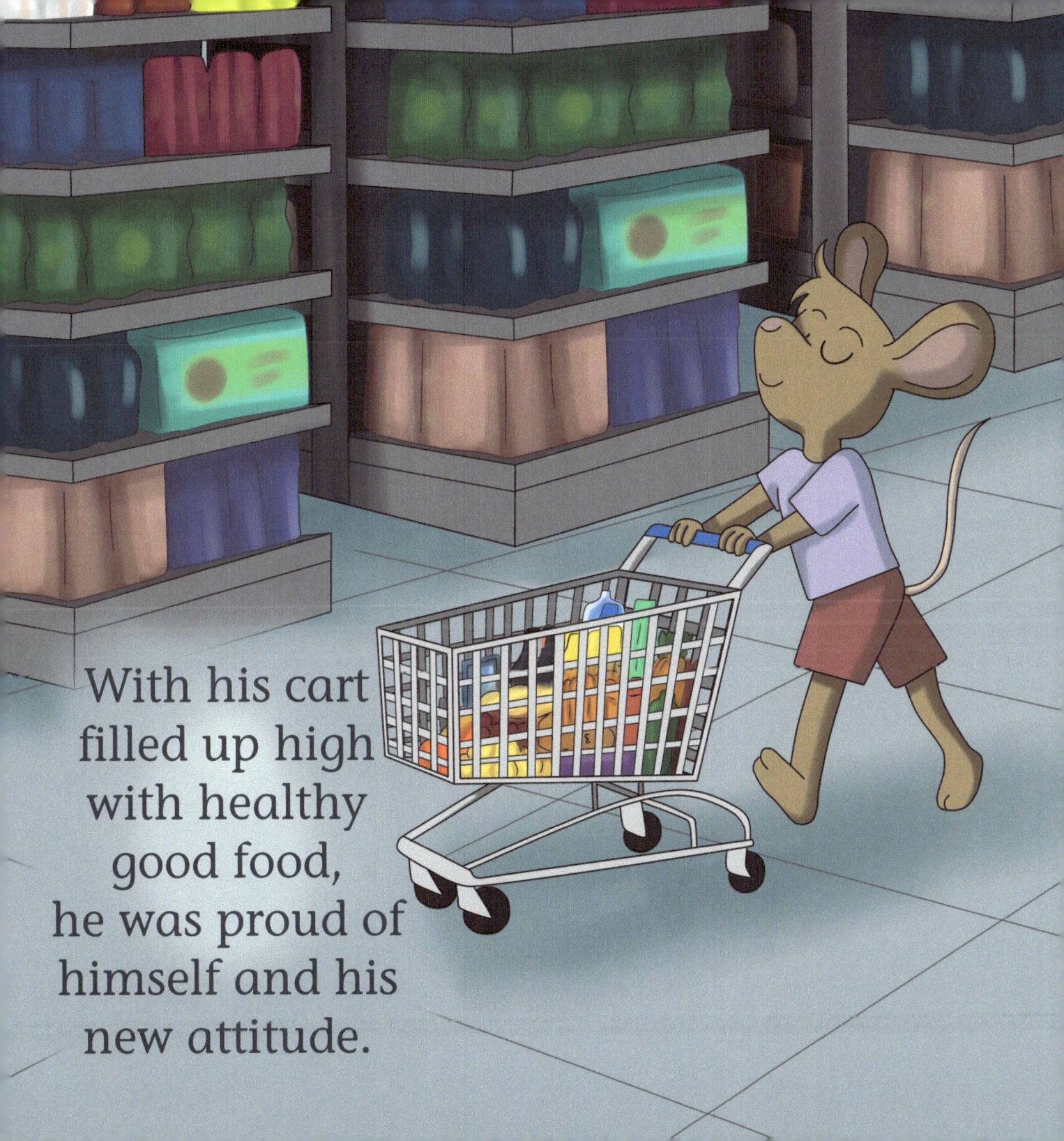

With his cart filled up high with healthy good food, he was proud of himself and his new attitude.

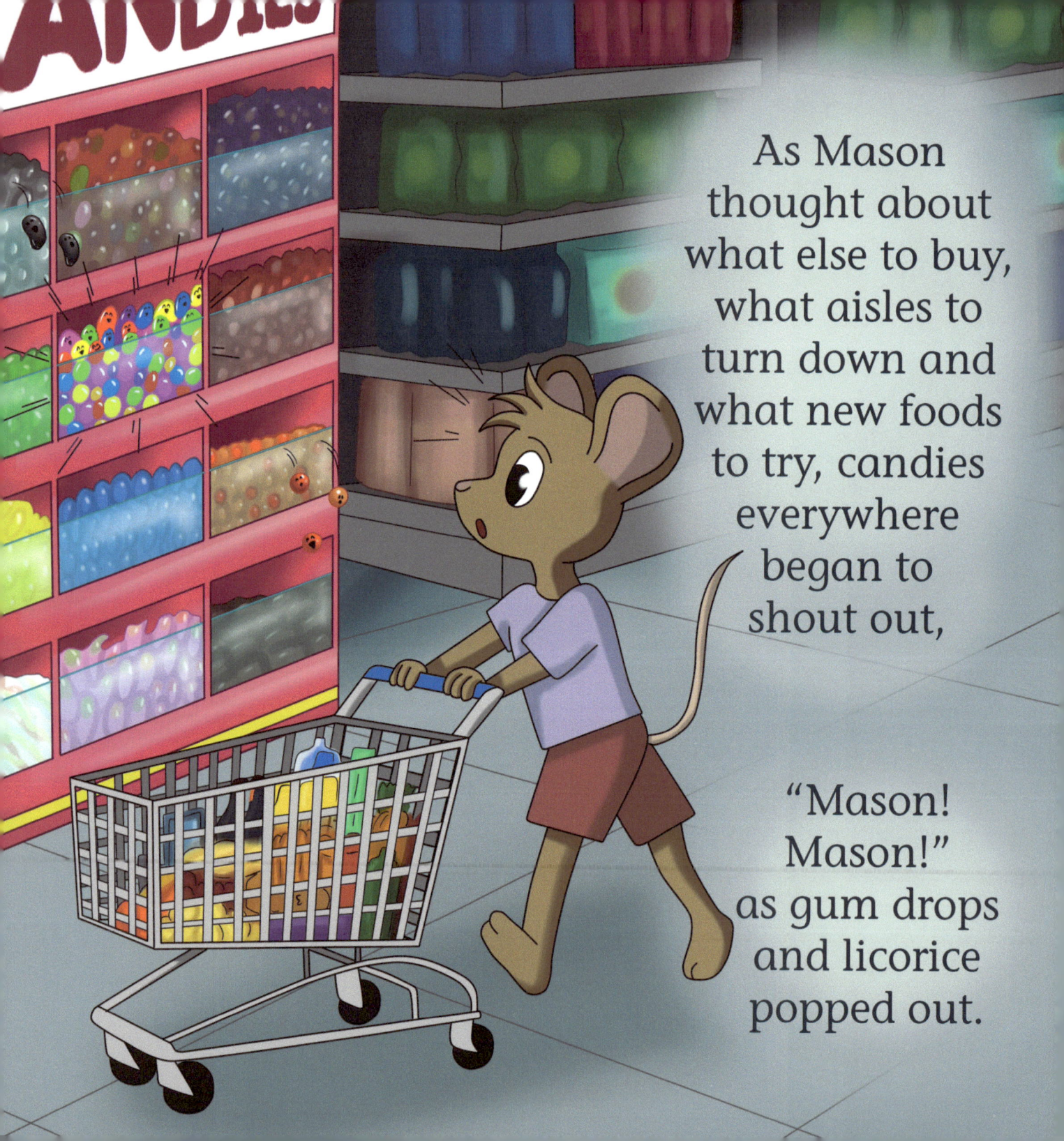

As Mason thought about what else to buy, what aisles to turn down and what new foods to try, candies everywhere began to shout out,

"Mason! Mason!" as gum drops and licorice popped out.

Jelly beans jumping all on their own
yelling, "Mason, Mason, please take us home!"
Red, black, and yellow, they all looked delicious
but Mason wanted something truly nutritious.

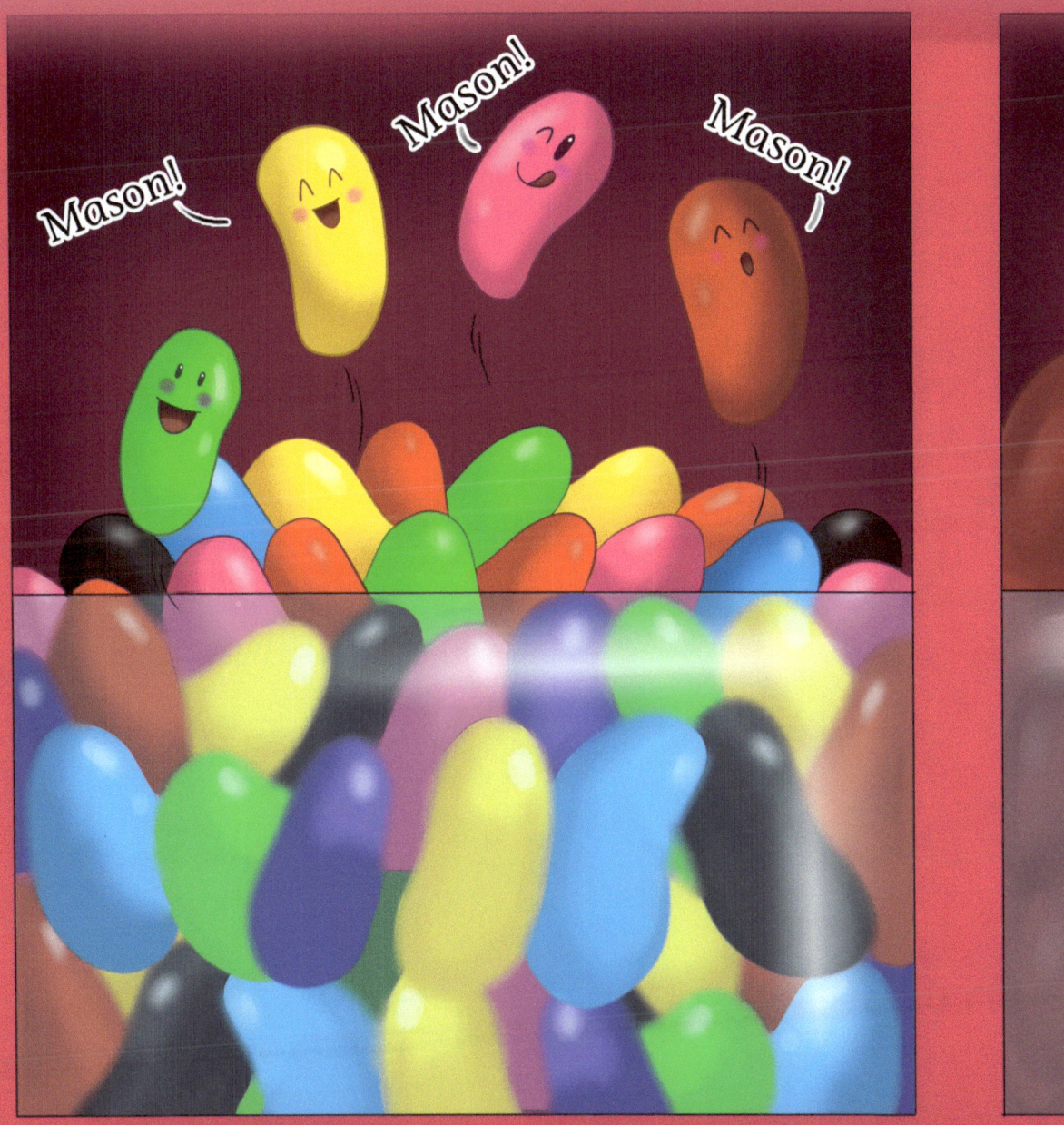

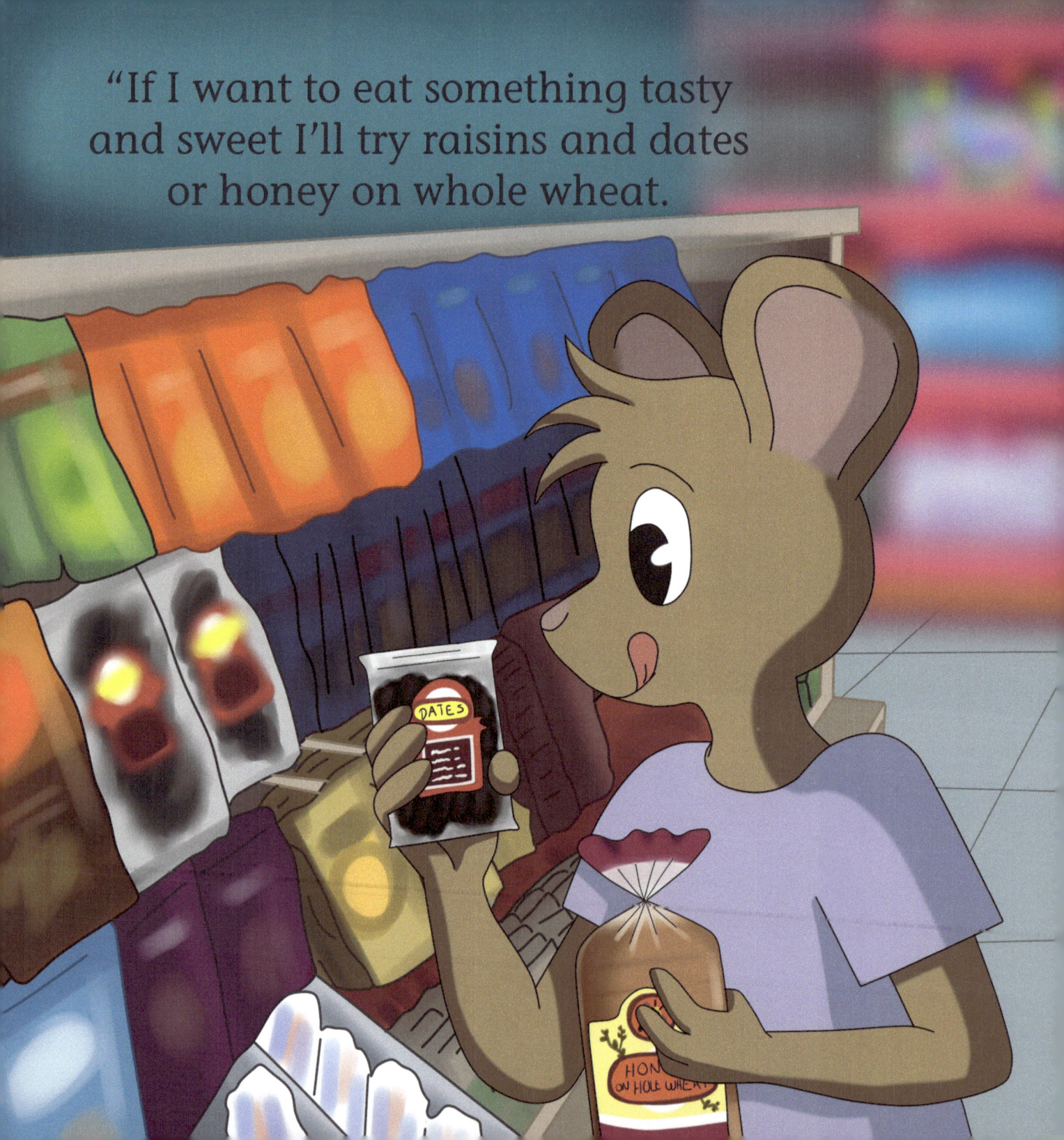

"If I want to eat something tasty and sweet I'll try raisins and dates or honey on whole wheat.

Carmel popcorn, well, once in a while. "Just a little bit will give me a smile!"

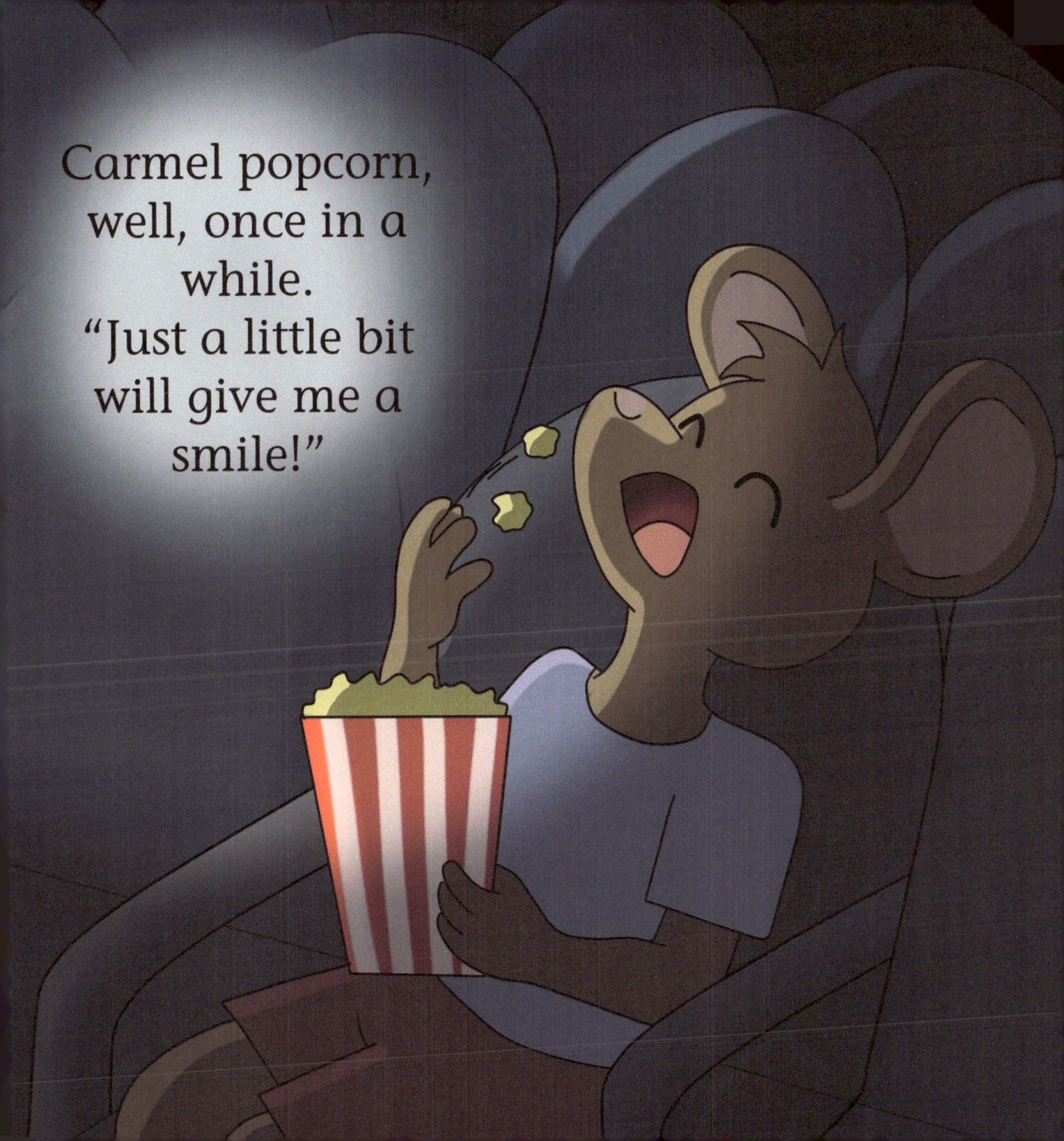

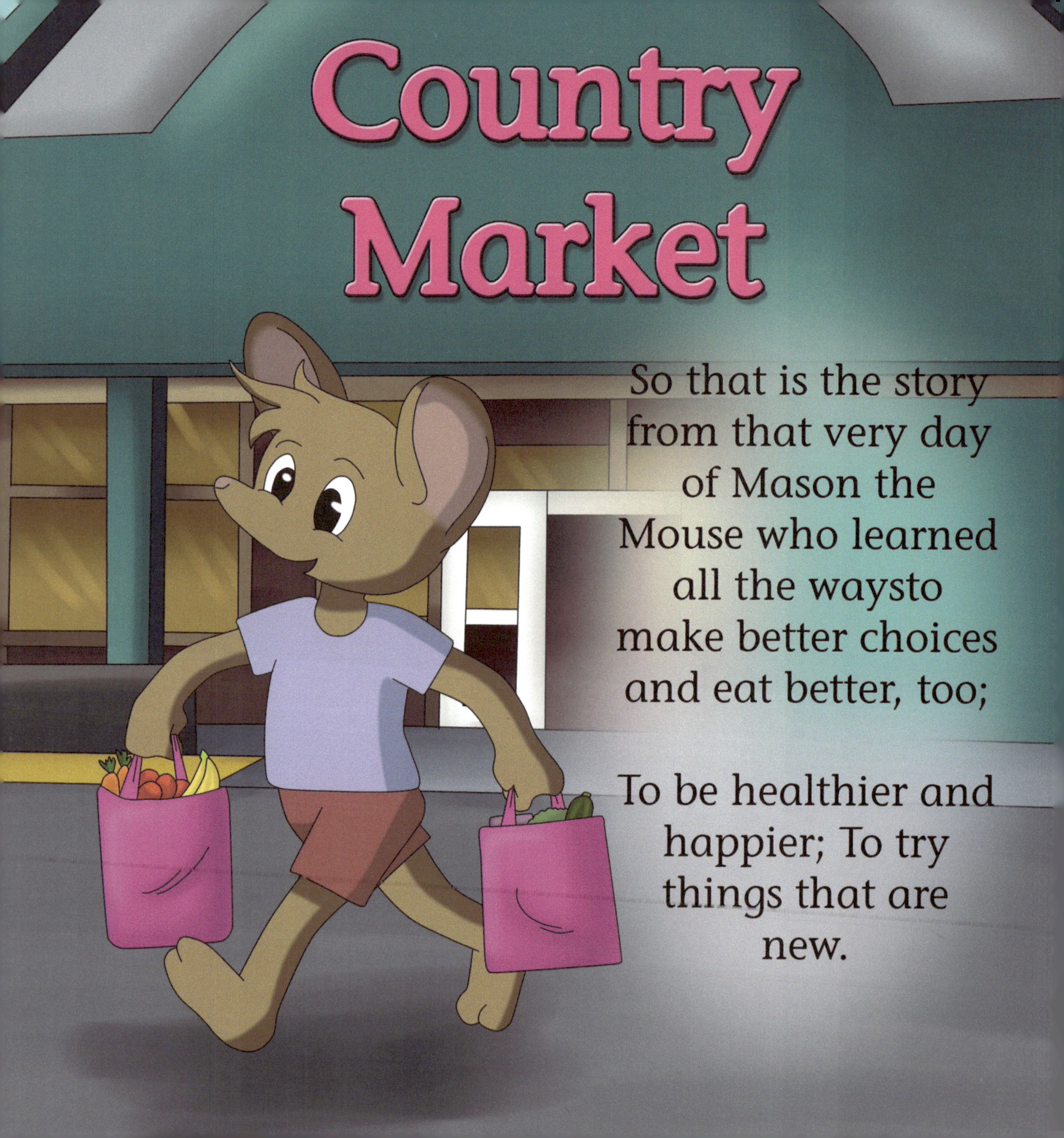

Country Market

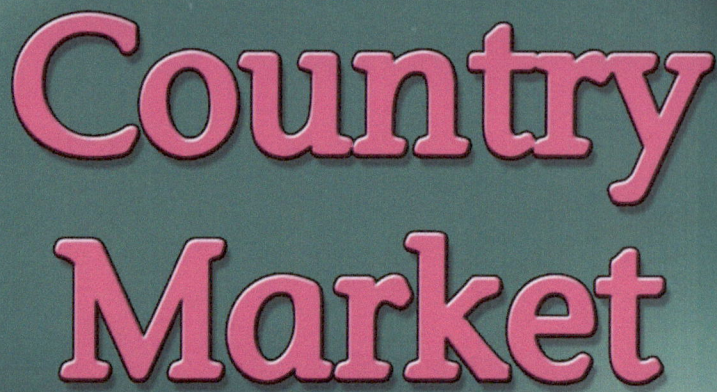

So that is the story from that very day of Mason the Mouse who learned all the ways to make better choices and eat better, too;

To be healthier and happier; To try things that are new.

Who is Ron Henderson?

Ron Henderson, AKA the Fitness King, is a renowned personal trainer, motivational speaker and writer who has been the premier personal fitness trainer in the Twin Cities for over 35 years. His expertise has landed him interviews with numerous newspapers, magazines, radio stations and TV programs. Ron is the author of What is it Worth for You to Become Physically Fit?, Fitness Economics, and Fitness and Faith: Balancing the Scales. He has hosted the cable TV show The King and the Kids which was geared to motivate all children to get up and move.

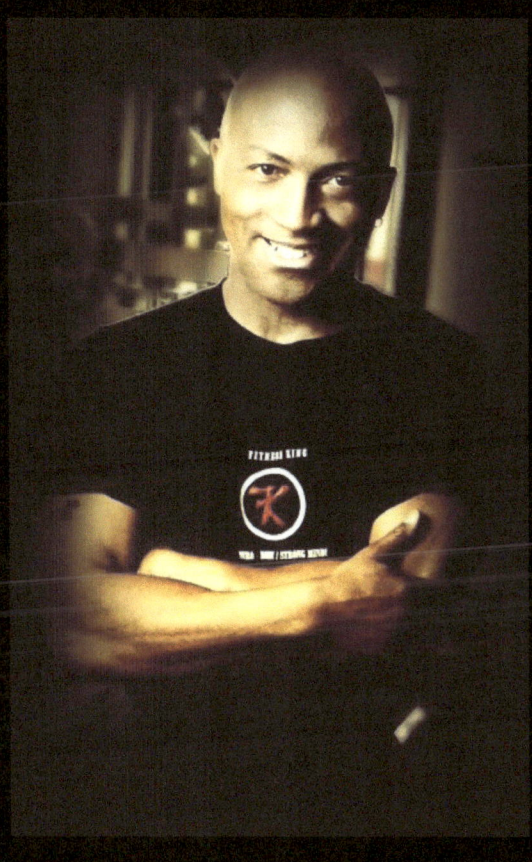